Keto Di
Beginners

Step-by-step Guide for Women Over 50 with Recipes For Rapid Weight Loss

By Jason Smith

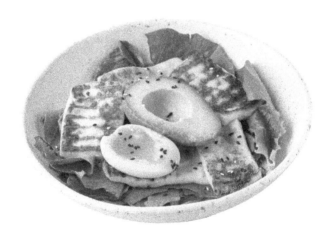

reparation, damages, or monetary loss due to the information herein, either directly or indirectly.

Respective authors own all copyrights not held by the publisher.

The information herein is offered for informational purposes solely and is universal as such. The presentation of the information is without a contract or any type of guarantee assurance.

The trademarks that are used are without any consent, and the publication of the trademark is without permission or backing by the trademark owner. All trademarks and brands within this book are for clarifying purposes only and are owned by the owners themselves, not affiliated with this document.

Contents

Chapter 1: Introduction to Ketogenic Diet 11

1.1.   Origin of Ketogenic Diet 14

1.2. Mechanism of Ketosis Diet 20

1.2.1. How does a Ketogenic Diet work? 21

1.2.   Myths about Ketogenic Diet 25

1.4. Benefits of Ketogenic Diet 34

1.4.1. Diabetes.. 35

1.4.2. Weight Loss.. 36

1.4.3. Cardiovascular Disease................................. 36

1.4.4. Epilepsy.. 37

1.4.5. Cancer.. 37

1.4.6. Alzheimer's disease 37

1.4.7. Neurological disorders 37

1.4.8. Reverse PCOS 38

1.4.9. Efficient against fighting with metabolic syndrome 38

Chapter 2: Menopause and Ketogenic Diet 40

2.1. Six ways to improve menopause through keto 42

Chapter 3: Do's and Don'ts of Ketogenic Diet.............................. 47

3.1. Do's of Keto diet 47

3.2. Don'ts of Keto Diet................................... 51

Chapter 4: Keto Meal Plan 65

4.2. Keto Diet grocery list 68

    4.2.1 List of Week 1 68

    4.2.2 List of Week 2 72

4.3. Keto Diet Pyramid 76

Chapter 5: Ketogenic diet meal recipes. 77

5.1. Recipes for breakfast 77

    1. Veggies and Parmesan with Sheet Pan Eggs 77

    2. Tomato Mozzarella Egg Muffins 78

    3. Cinnamon & Almond Porridge 79

    4. Crispy Chai Waffles 80

    5. Sheet Pan Eggs with Ham and Pepper Jack 82

5.2 Recipes for lunch 83

    1. Three Meat & Cheese Sandwich 83

    2. Kebabs of Beef and Pepper 84

    3. Chicken tenders with Coconut 85

    4. Ham, Egg & Cheese Sandwich 86

    5.Curried Chicken Soup 88

5.3. Recipes for dinner 90

    1.   Baked Lamb Chops with Asparagus 90

    2.   Kebabs of Lemon Chicken with Vegetables 91

    3.   Spicy Chicken Enchilada Casserole 92

    4.   White Cheddar Broccoli Chicken Casserole 93

    5.   Stuffed Bell Peppers Bacon 94

5.4. Keto dessert recipes 96

    1.   Cashew Macadamia Fat Bomb Bars 96

2. Coconut Truffles from Cocoa 97

3. Chocolate Sun butter 98

4. Coco-Almond Bomb Bars of Fat 99

5. Chocolate-Dipped Pecan Fat Bombs 100

Conclusion 101

Introduction

The present accessibility of data implies all that we need to think about anything is readily available, or with one swipe. That same accessibility can often leave you with an excess of knowledge. How would you interpret everything and decide whether intermittent fasting and keto are ideal for you? That is the objective of this book. We did a profound plunge on such lifestyles and analyzed the benefits such practices implemented on their own and combined so you'll cut straight to the chase and acquire started on your intermittent keto venture. Before you set out making changes, approach this as you would any recipe, read the directions from start to end. Ensure you comprehend not exactly how to do intermittent fasting and cook keto-accommodating suppers but the science behind it. Perusing all the starting material will make the progress to this new way of life simpler and help you see the perfect results at the end. Enticing as it is very easy maybe to jump directly to the Meal Plan and recipes. Remember that a strong base is a way to progress. The words between this presentation and the plans give the blocks and mortar to assemble a strong beginning.

It drives us to a decision to vigorously alter our physical body weight or figure because we are not satisfied with our normal body shape or height. Any effort in the name of weight loss is referred to as dieting. A study said that Americans normally invest more than $40 billion a year on dieting and diet-related items. It is often recorded that at some point in time or typically after the age of 50, 60% of women are trying to lose weight. There are too many common methods of dieting or shaping the form or size of the body of which the method of a ketogenic diet (in the short-term, keto) is so well established. A ketogenic diet is a meal with an appropriate protein intake, low in carbohydrates, and heavy in fat consumption. Typically, `ketogenic diet is viewed as a daunting regimen to adopt. It becomes a convenient routine, however, with practice and an understanding of what the diet targets are to attain. The underlying goal is to shift the main fuel supply of the body from carbohydrates such as sugar and bread to fats. It can be done by increasing the consumption of fats and significantly reducing the intake of carbohydrates. The actual effort is that the meal portion is so restrictive like all foodstuffs eaten must be weighed out to a 10th of a gram in meal preparations, and the one who diets may not eat anything which is not "recommended" by the dietician. The level of carbohydrates permitted is very small so that even the minor quantity of sugar in most liquid or chewable pills will avert the diet from working.

Chapter 1: Introduction to Ketogenic Diet

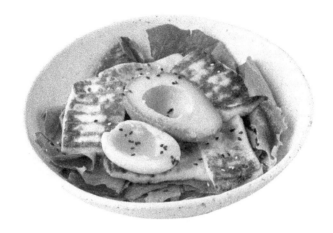

Before conversing the particulars of a ketogenic diet, it is useful to discuss some preliminary information. This contains a general overview of a ketogenic diet procedure as well as the history of its growth, equally for medical situations as well as for fat loss. Intermittent fasting and ketosis, (Known as IF and Keto) target the core system of how you consume food or the selections you make with every meal. Fulfilled properly, keto is life changes, and lasting solutions for a healthy, happy, and smart you.

Carbohydrates on the surface, are a rapid, often fast, and inexpensive form of nutrition to get power throughout the day. Recall all those grab-and-go snacks we associate with our breakfast. Those granola bars, smoothies with fruit-filled, muffins. We resume our mornings with carbs, and as the day progresses, we keep piling them on. Only because anything works doesn't mean that it's the right way to do it. To keep us alive, the tissues and cells that make up our bodies require energy to perform daily functions. There are two main sources from which the foods we consume will derive nutrition. Carbohydrates, which transform into glucose, are one source of nutrition. It is the latest current model that is adopted by most of us. However, there is an alternate fuel, and an interesting one: fat. Yeah, the very thing that you've been advised to restrict your whole life might just be the niche you need to improve your metabolism. When our bodies metabolize food and break down fatty acids, organic compounds, called ketones, are released. To keep our cells and muscles functioning, ketones serve as electricity. Throughout your life, you have undoubtedly used the word "metabolism," but do you know exactly what it means? The word refers to the chemical reactions needed to remain alive in any living organism. Of course, considering the intricacies of the human body, our metabolism is anything but simply gives the complexities to the human body. Our bodies are at work endlessly, even when we sleep, our cells actively construct and rebuild themselves. They need to be able to draw energy from our bodies. One way to fuel our metabolism is glucose, which is what carbohydrates are broken down into after we consume them. As the main energy source, our new dietary recommendations concentrate on carbohydrates. Factor in the additional sugar that we consume and the recommended regular portions of berries, starchy vegetables, grains, and protein sources dependent on plants (e.g., beans), and our bodies do not lack glucose. The concern with this energy use paradigm is that it leaves us on one of those wheels spinning like hamsters. We burn energy but get nowhere, especially if we eat more carbohydrates than our bodies can use in a day's work. But that's the other source of energy that I've mentioned: fat. How specifically does it work? Is it feasible to utilize this alternate type of fuel to enable our body to burn energy more effectively, for greater overall health benefits? We're back to the old notion of what you eat is what you are. Except now think about the principal theory instead of as you burn what you eat. It is when it falls into action for ketosis. Switching to a low-carb, high-fat, moderate-protein diet helps the body to reach a state of ketosis, in which you metabolize fat, allowing ketones to be emitted to power the functions of our intricate inner workings. Through the liver when fatty acids are broken down, it produces ketones. It is about equilibrium to maintain a state of ketosis, but not the sort you are accustomed to when it comes to eating. Our present food pyramid, which instructs us to eat an enormous quantity of foods abundant in carbohydrates for energy, turns out to be upside down. Fats at the top make up 60 to 80 percent of your diet; protein in the center at 20 to 30 percent; and carbs (actual glucose in disguise) at the bottom, making for just 5 to 10 percent of your everyday eating schedule. A more effective plan for feeding your body.

1.1. Origin of Ketogenic Diet

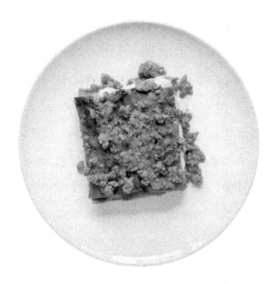

In the first place, we need to discuss the brief history of a ketogenic diet from where it came. a ketogenic diet is not at all a new treatment. In all over history it has been acknowledged that if a person with epilepsy stops eating or fasts, their seizures usually stop. In the earlier time, numerous nutritional "treatments" for epilepsy were introduced, and such cures included the increase or restraint of almost every ingredient such as vegetables, animals, and minerals. Though, fasting or starving as a cure for seizures or attacks was less recognized. Fasting is the only calming measure against epilepsy documented in some researches. Research in the 5th century BC, conducted on a person who had been seized by epileptic fits after having smeared himself before the fire in a bath. Completely abstinence from diet and drink was suggested, and the cure was effective. In the early 20th century, the medicinal use of a ketogenic diet appeared as a tactic to mimic the biochemical effects of fasting. In starting of the 20th century, some physicians present the first scientific research on the importance of fasting in epilepsy. They said the attacks were less during treatment.

Now, let's take a look at history in detail. In the past, several epilepsy nutritional "cures" have been advocated, and those therapies have involved the surplus or limitation of every ingredient (animals, minerals, or vegetables). Additionally, while fasting has been accepted for more than two and a half thousand years as a cure for many illnesses, fasting is less recognized as a remedy for seizures. The only preventive intervention against epilepsy registered in the Hippocratic collection is fasting. Five centuries later, fasting was recorded in Biblical times as a treatment for epilepsy. Mark tells the story of the Jesus treating an epileptic child in a quote from the King James Translation of the Bible (Huisjen, 2000).

In 1911, a pair of Parisian doctors, Gulep and Marie, reported the first modern use of starvation as a cure for epilepsy. They treated 20 children and adults with epilepsy and confirmed that aftercare, seizures became less frequent, although no clear specifics were provided. Contemporary fasting reports from the United States were often reported at the beginning of the 20th century: the first was a study on an osteopathic doctor's patient of Battle Creek's

Dr. Hugh W. Conklin, Michigan; and the second involved Bernarr Macfadden (Freeman et al., 1994). Macfadden was a physical exercise guru/cultist in the early part of the 20th century and a publishing master. He instructed readers about how to physically improve themselves, how to preserve their wellbeing, and how to live with the disease. Every issue of his journal, Physical Culture, held articles about sickly men and women who, by proper diet and exercise, became fit, strong, and attractive. The magazine's distribution had surpassed 500,000 by the close of World War I. Macfadden believed that fasting could relieve and heal just about any condition, including epilepsy, for 3 days to 3 weeks. He had been nationally known, and as part of a plan to be named as the first Health Secretary in 1931, he sought to ingratiate himself with a presidential contender, Franklin D. Roosevelt (Wilkinson, 1997). Dr. Conklin started as Macfadden's assistant and implemented his fasting approach to cure multiple illnesses. It was the fasting procedure of Dr. Conklin to cure epilepsy and the consequences that attracted the interest of another leader in epilepsy science, H. Rawle Geyelin, a New York-Presbyterian Hospital endocrinologist. Dr. Geyelin first recorded his knowledge of fasting as a cure for epilepsy at the American Medical Association Conference in 1921. The leader who records the cognitive development that could arise with fasting was Dr. Geyelin. Dr. Geyelin's lecture was witnessed by Drs. W.G. and Stanley Cobb. Harvard's Lennox. The popularity of Dr. Conklin's fasting outcomes spread steadily and by 1941 it had acquired attention from the Montreal Neurologic Institute in the textbook of Penfield and Erickson on epilepsy. Drs. in the starting of the 1920s, at Harvard Medical School, Cobb and Lennox started researching the impact of hunger on epilepsy therapy. They became the first to notice that there was usually an increase in seizures after 2-3 days. Lennox reported that seizure regulation happened by a transition in the metabolism of the body and that the mere lack of food or starch deprivation in the body caused the body to burn acid-forming fat. Two decisive discoveries were made in 1921. Woodyatt observed that acetone and beta-hydroxybutyric acid occur from malnutrition or a diet comprising too low a carbohydrate proportion and too high a fat proportion in a typical topic (Woodyatt, 1921). At the same time, Dr. Wilder at Mayo Clinic indicated that if ketonemia was created through some methods, the effects of fasting might be achieved (Wilder, 1921). In a sequence of patients with epilepsy, wilder suggested that a ketogenic diet (KD) be attempted. The diet could be as productive as fasting and could be sustained for a much longer period, he suggested. Wilder later published at Mayo Clinic on patients treated with the ketone-producing diet and invented the word "ketogenic diet. In 1925, Peterman at the Clinic named Mayo, eventually reported the KD formula identical to that used today: 1 g of protein per kilogram of body weight in infants, 10-15 g of carbohydrates per day, and the rest of the calories in fat. The value of training caregiver's diet management before discharge, diet individualization, and near follow-up was reported by Peterman. Also, Peterman observed shifts in behavior and cognitive symptoms that followed the KD. These initial findings were soon accompanied by reports from Harvard and McQuarrie and Keith at Mayo Clinic from Talbot et al. In nearly every detailed textbook about epilepsy in kids that came in 1941 and in1980, the use of KD was documented. Most of the material in the book included complete chapters explaining the diet, how to start it, or the ways to measure meal plans. The KD was frequently used in the 1920s, also in the 1930s. In 1972 Livingston, at Johns Hopkins Hospital, published in his textbook on the outcomes of the diet of over 1,000 epilepsy children he had followed in previous decades (Livingston, 1972). He indicated that 52% had absolute regulation of the seizures and a further 27% had increased control.

In the year 1938, diphenylhydantoin was identified by Putnam & Merritt, the interest of researchers moved from the KD's action mode and usefulness to experimental antiepileptic medications. The modern age of epilepsy drug therapy has started and the KD has faded away. In an attempt to render the classic KD more palatable, the medium-chain triglyceride oil diet was developed by Dr. Peter Huttenlocher at the University of Chicago in 1971, enabling some foods to be less limited. The KD was used less and lesser as new antiepileptic medications were available. It was anticipated that this branched fatty acid chain would treat kids formerly put on the regime to treat Lennox-Gastaut syndrome seizures after the advent of sodium valproate and the regimen could no longer be explained. Pediatric neurologists were encouraged to conclude that the rationally designed antiepileptic drugs were the anticipation for the future. Few infants were put on KD, which culminated in fewer dietitians being qualified to use the diet. A scarcity of adequately qualified dietitians means that, without accurate measurement, the KD was frequently applied, contributing to the impression that the diet was unsuccessful. The usage of KD was often based on the understanding of the public. From 1970 to 2000, the usage of KD declined dramatically and PubMed listed just two to eight publications a year. However, when NBC-Dateline TV's broadcast a documentary on the procedure, this shifted drastically when the KD gained mainstream media coverage. A dramatic increase in PubMed publications totaling over 40 a year since then has corresponded with this. This television show was focused on the real tale of Charlie, a 2-year-old child with intractable generalized epilepsy who applied for treatment at Johns Hopkins Hospital out of desperation. Dr. Freeman and Ms. Millicent Kelly (the same dietitian who collaborated with Dr. Livingston) met him and welcomed him to KD. He soon became seizure-free, and his father founded the Charlie Foundation. Informational videos for parents and educational videos for doctors and dietitians regarding KD are disseminated by this foundation. It also helped finance the initial publishing of The Introduction to a Ketogenic Diet: The Epilepsy Diet Cure (Freeman et al., 1994). In 1997, Charlie's father directed the film "First Do No Harm" featuring Meryl Streep, which appeared on national TV. The Foundation sponsored the first multicenter prospective analysis of the KD's effectiveness (Vining et al., 1998).

In recent years, the KD has undergone a re-emergence and modern clinical trials have validated the therapy as being substantially successful (Freeman et al., 1998). KD is currently accessible in over 45 countries around the world (Kossoff &

McGrogan, 2005). However, when this therapy is used by pediatric neurologists, physician perception still has a significant influence. Two recent expert opinion surveys, one conducted in the United States and one conducted in Europe, revealed that KD was the next-to-the-last or last option for almost all childhood epilepsy treatment. Furthermore, a recent study of child neurologists also ranked KD as a therapy that they typically used last, with many not using it at all. There is still a great deal of work to be done to improve the perception of the usefulness of KD, a treatment that compares favorably with other new treatments introduced for the treatment of childhood epilepsy.

Almost a century has passed since the initial use of KD, and many more therapies for children with epilepsy are now available. In the United States, KD has a rich history and continues to be used to treat refractory childhood epilepsy. At almost all major children's hospitals, it is available. Our understanding of the scientific research of this unique therapy has evolved dramatically, resulting in this first international conference dedicated to the KD. A better understanding of the scientific basis of this unique dietary therapy will continue to rise with this renewed scientific interest, resulting in improved epilepsy treatment for all children. This will be an appropriate legacy for the KD.

1.2. Mechanism of Ketosis Diet

A ketogenic diet follows a starving or abstaining state by stopping the body when it requires carbohydrates to function normally, and driving it to metabolize fats. Once the fat is metabolized, ketone bodies are formed. It is the production of the ketone bodies which seems to play a vital role in the accomplishment of a ketogenic diet. When the body starts to produce ketone bodies, it is denoted as the body is in ketosis. It typically takes 3 – 5 days for the body to go into ketosis, once a person starting the diet. Ketosis is easily recognized, because the ketones can be noticed in the urine, and can be recognized by a specific smell of the person's breathing. The prophylactic characteristics of a ketogenic diet form up with time and it may take quite a few weeks before the full outcome of a ketogenic diet is attained.

1.2.1. How does a Ketogenic Diet work?

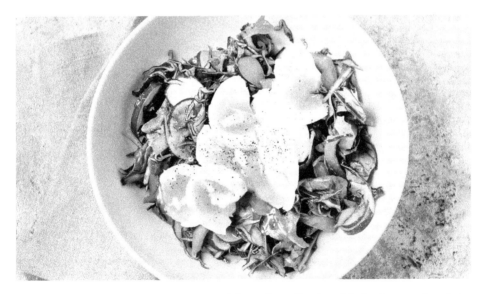

The food we consume provides the fuel which is required to support the body for everyday activity and also provides that material that our body needs to grow. The body is built to use three primary fuels, including carbohydrates, fats, and proteins, unlike vehicles that can only run on oil. Carbohydrates are the primary ingredient of predominantly plant-derived sugars, starch, and wheat.

There are two broad categories of fats: saturated fats, such as butter, mostly derived from livestock, and unsaturated fats, such as corn oil, mostly derived from plants. Protein, finally, comes mostly from plants and is expressed by beef and fish. The above is a large generalization and there are several variants, such as nuts having more than 50% fat. Carbohydrates, fats, and proteins all undergo the same form of chemical reaction, like carbon dioxide and water, for the air we breathe to generate nutrition for the body and waste materials. This is the same response that is noticed when an automobile engine consumes oil or when heat burns wood or coal, etc. While all three fuels in the body are metabolized in the same manner. Carbohydrates, accompanied by fats and proteins, are preferentially utilized. Carbohydrates are used preferentially since in most individuals they are typically readily accessible, and the body will easily metabolize them for energy. Before an athletic performance to have additional energy, athletes sometimes consume some kind of high carbohydrate snack. Carbohydrates are usually utilized just a few hours after they are ingested, which is one explanation why we feed so much. Unused carbohydrates are processed or transformed into fat in the form of glycogen in the liver. The primary function of fats, by comparison, is to store energy. To brace for winter, livestock fattens up. The body usually retains the fats we consume, so the body can break down the fat stores and use them as energy if there are not enough carbohydrates accessible. Fats are metabolized somewhat gradually and it would usually require a day or two to use the fat content of a meal. This explains why people feel fuller as opposed to a low carbohydrate meal after a fatty meal. Protein, the third nutrient, is mainly used to build and replenish body materials; any surplus protein is metabolized or excreted as fuel. The body may continue to break down muscle to metabolize the protein for fuel if carbohydrate and fat reserves are exhausted. The proportion (by weight) of the three fuels used would be around 5-15% protein, 10-20% fat, and 65-85%

the carbohydrate in a traditional western diet. The body can retain some extra "fuel" as fat, or excrete it. The amount of fats in a ketogenic diet, on the other side, is substantially improved and the proportion of carbohydrates is drastically decreased. It is therefore important to monitor the overall food consumption since if the body is provided excess, it would preferentially dump the fats to revert to its preferred fuel balance. The body is forced to metabolize fat in favor of carbohydrates by limiting its overall caloric intake.

By refusing the body the carbohydrate it needs to function properly, thus pressuring it to metabolize fat, a ketogenic diet mimics a hunger or fasting condition. Ketone bodies are shaped when the fat is metabolized. It is the formation of ketone bodies that tends to play a key role in the effectiveness of a ketogenic diet. It is referred to as the body being in ketosis as the body starts making ketone bodies. Since initiating the diet, it typically takes 3 to 5 days for the body to done ketosis. Ketosis is quickly recognizable since the ketones in the urine can be identified and can be recognized by the distinctive smell of the breath of the person. The prophylactic effects of the ketogenic diet grow with time and it will take many weeks for a ketogenic diet to have its maximum impact.

1.2. Myths about Ketogenic Diet

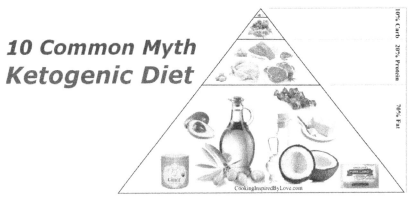

Low Carb High Fat Ketogenic Food Pyramid

A ketogenic diet is presently trending as the greatest diet for weight reduction till now. It's rich in fat and a low-carbohydrate diet that forms ketones. The effect of the breakdown of fats in the liver to be used as energy. With a keto diet numerous things are being said that is correct, but a lot of things that aren't so factual as well.

We will expose 14 myths about the keto diet below, including those linked with what to

suppose throughout the transition period, finest ratios of macros, and possible benefits

like good weight loss and mental comprehension help.

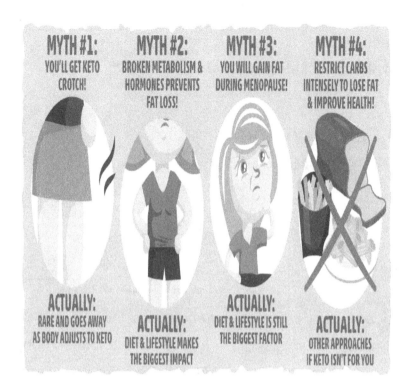

MYTH #1: YOU'LL GET KETO CROTCH!

MYTH #2: BROKEN METABOLISM & HORMONES PREVENTS FAT LOSS!

MYTH #3: YOU WILL GAIN FAT DURING MENOPAUSE!

MYTH #4: RESTRICT CARBS INTENSELY TO LOSE FAT & IMPROVE HEALTH!

ACTUALLY: RARE AND GOES AWAY AS BODY ADJUSTS TO KETO

ACTUALLY: DIET & LIFESTYLE MAKES THE BIGGEST IMPACT

ACTUALLY: DIET & LIFESTYLE IS STILL THE BIGGEST FACTOR

ACTUALLY: OTHER APPROACHES IF KETO ISN'T FOR YOU

1. The Rich in fat, rich in protein diet is Keto.

A keto diet isn't especially abundant in protein, unlike another common low-carb diet. In reality, when on a keto diet, protein consumption always must be "adequate" because this helps you to switch to ketosis and remain there. In general, so abundant protein in the diet can contribute to few of the protein being transformed to glucose until ingested, and this will be detrimental when it is about to retaining relatively low amounts of glucose. Then what proportion of protein are you going to need? A typical guideline for a ketogenic diet is to receive around 75% of the everyday calories from fat sources (for instance oils or fatty meat cuts), 5% from carbs, and 20% from protein (take or give a little is depending on the dieter). Rich-protein, low-carb diets, on the other hand, can include having 30 to 35 % (or sometimes more) of regular protein calories.

2. A Keto diet is solely a weight reduction diet.

Without any doubt over that, a ketogenic diet would promote successful weight loss. Although this does not mean that a keto diet should not be implemented to support a healthier weight if one of the goals is not good weight management. By widely encouraging metabolic fitness, for example, healthy body composition, the effects of keto will achieve a good degree of balanced mental results beyond weight advantages. Will you gain weight from a keto diet? It is perhaps possible, particularly if you do not properly embrace the diet and may not have ketosis. It is commonly accepted that if calorie intake is lower than needed by someone, Regardless of the type of diet anyone follows, weight loss will always a result in fact, from where

the calories come.

The key point? If we eat more calories daily than we do, if the source of calories is protein or fats, then you may notice the scale creeping up.

3. Claims for health care are simply claims. There's also no research.

This can't have been farther from the facts! In 1920, Johns Hopkins Medical Center doctors first established a ketogenic diet. At that moment, hundreds of experiments have studied the

impact of the diet.

4. You can't perform the workout on Keto.

For everyone, counting those on a ketogenic diet, exercising is helpful. At the start, during the workout, you feel that your energy decreases, but this would disperse as the body changes.

A ketogenic diet does not appear to trigger any loss in efficiency for most individuals, particularly in the middle of high-intensity workouts; in reality, some report getting even extra energy because the fats for fuel can be used by the body effectively. Make sure you eat sufficient calories in total and lots of fat to sustain your exercises. And if you still fail to remain active when on a diet, consider raising your carbohydrates, a little and/or attempting a more "improved ketogenic diet."

5. On the ketogenic diet and keto lifestyle, you will lose body mass.

On a keto diet, will you grow muscle? There's some proof that you can, yeah. This is how it might be a perfect way to help muscle building and boost resilience by mixing a ketogenic diet with strength-training. And keto diet does not, on its own, induce more muscle mass loss like any other diet, until you reduce calories.

6. The same thing goes with ketoacidosis & ketosis.

The two of them are very distinct and would not be mistaken. Ketoacidosis is observed as a severe diabetic problem that arises when excess ketones are produced by the body (or we can say blood acids). However, ketosis is a physiological condition in which much of the food for the body is produced by fat.

7. During their transition period, everybody faces such things.

Each person responds very differently to a ketogenic diet, so it's difficult to judge

what you might come across. Some persons smoothly move into ketosis, while others do not.

Although these encounters may at first be unpleasant, it is usual for them to go out after one

or two weeks, so be optimistic. Through eating a "well balanced" ketogenic diet, consume

adequate water, sodium, and electrolytes (such as magnesium or potassium, like as from a

Ketogenic Multi and vegetables), fiber, you will further minimize the discomfort you feel,

might be in supplementing with exogenous ketones (which is the form of Keto Fire).

8. On the keto, you will still have little sugar.

Some feel that their vitality and focus gets a boost as they adapt to be in ketosis. Ketones are doing a better job by supplying a constant supply of food to the brain, but staying in ketosis (and adding keto-friendly vitamins) will benefit by encouraging mental clarity, concentration, and a healthy mindset.

9. You can only remain for a brief amount of time on the keto.

In general speaking, it is advised that if you start a keto diet the first time, you continue the diet for around 2 to 3 months, and then stop for a while. Offer your body some weeks to adjust and, if it fits well for you, hop right on the ketogenic diet. Depending on how you feel, you might want to comfortably move in or out of the ketosis for several months or years. You can still contact a health provider, though. A ketogenic diet has no fixed time limit; it's just about finding out what fits better for you with your routine and objectives.

10. Occasionally, you can cheat while on keto

It may not be reasonable to ask you to adhere 100% to a keto diet. But dissimilar other diets, where it is possible to allow "cheat days" to offer you a pause and also promote your metabolism, your ketosis might shift out while cheating on the keto diet. If it's deliberate, this must not be a concern. As far as we know it's going on and you change your diet consequently, cycling a ketogenic diet out here is all right. If you notice that because of "cheating" and growing your carb consumption, you are no longer in ketosis, so by increasing your fats and reducing your carbohydrates, you will easily take some days to get back in.

11. On a keto diet, you can consume some form of fat, equivalent to common low-carb diets.

Because a keto diet isn't just about good weight loss, as compared to any forms of fatty foodstuffs, healthy fats are promoted. Many persons on a keto diet, for example, tend to eliminate high-fat fatty meat items such as bacon or pork, poor-quality sausage, and salami.

Continue to "eat clean" if you need the best out of the diet; skip trans-fats, refined goods produced from poor-quality vegetable oils, most fried foods, fast food, cheeses, and meats of questionable quality. Choose safe and cold-pressed oils (such as coconut oil or natural olive), butter, grass-fed and beef, pasture-raised livestock, wild-caught seafood, and cage-free eggs to acquire your fats from safe sources.

12. For women and men, Keto is the same.

Overall, compared with males, women incline to be more susceptible to dietary shifts and weight. It's always feasible for the women to adopt a keto diet successfully and, if they prefer, to observe intermittent fasting, however, they can do so more cautiously.

In addition to a ketogenic diet, it is advised that women concentrate on consuming a nutritious, alkaline diet, ensuring they include plenty of vegetables that are non-starchy to ensure that they receive adequate nutrients & electrolytes. Ideally, the diet can be approached in different steps, initially concentrating on full alkaline foods before including the keto component & fasting. Women can, therefore, as far as possible, decrease such causes of tension and still, pay attention to their bodies. If you are a woman adopting a keto diet, do concentrate on how your outlook & energy are affected by exercise, and what amount of sleep you get every night, the exposure of sunlight you get, the consumption of caffeine alcohol, etc.

13. When on a keto diet, intermittent fasting must take place.

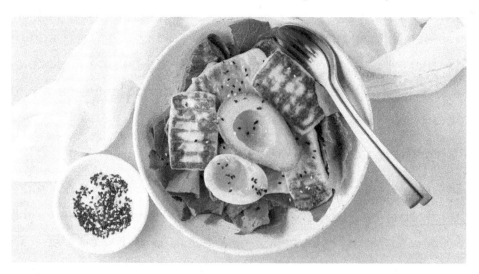

During a keto diet, intermittent fasting (known as IMF) is recommended and can help speed up outcomes (like detoxification and moving towards the weight loss goals), although it is not a necessity for ketosis to be reached or sustained. When adopting a keto diet, many individuals observe IMF to be simpler as ketosis is proven to help minimize cravings and to help sustain a regular, balanced appetite. If you are a bit hungry, not just because during a keto diet you consume plenty of gratifying fats, fiber from vegetables, and moderate protein, it happens due to ketones which help to curb appetite, so you will notice that fasting will not be

 tough as it would otherwise be.

14. While on keto, you can't consume alcohol.

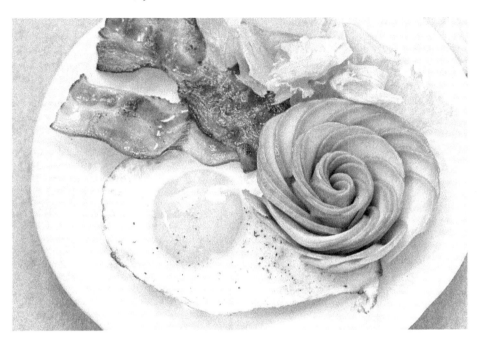

Although on the ketogenic diet, some people still prefer to drink alcohol in a balanced amount, particularly hard liquor & organic red wine. The aim is to sustain a small amount of alcohol consumption and to drink alcohol with a portion of food containing lots of fat and a certain amount of protein.

Beverages that are rich in carbs and sugar are not healthy options, such as sugar blended drinks and most breweries. If consuming alcohol allows sugar levels of blood to increase too high, and it makes it too tough to remain in ketosis, so to make a keto diet work for you, you may need to limit or eliminate alcohol.

1.4. Benefits of Ketogenic Diet

The ketogenic regimen is encircled by different controversies. Supporters of the ketogenic diet state that it is a phenomenal diet whereas rivals criticize the diet because of misconceptions about the functioning involved. As with so many questions of controversies, the truth is somewhere in between. Like most dietetic methods, a ketogenic diet has also almost no disadvantages but numerous benefits, which are as under.

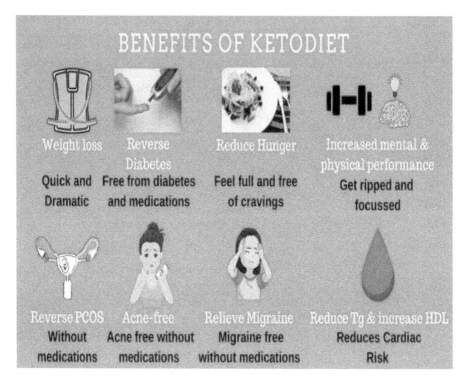

Let's have a peek at the carbohydrate pathway before exploring the advantages of the Ketogenic diet. Carbohydrates are absorbed and stored easily. Digestion begins in the mouth, as soon as the food is chewed, amylase (Such enzymes that digest carbohydrates) in the saliva now performing on the carbohydrates. In the stomach, carbohydrates are more broken down and are straightaway absorbed, once it goes into the small intestines. Carbohydrates immediately buildup the sugar level in the blood. This encourages the instant release of insulin.

High sugar level generates the release of high levels of insulin. This hormone causes the sugar to be deposited instantly in the body tissues to reduce the level of blood. Those issues can be insulin resistance when it is continually exposed to it at high levels. As the body tends to speedily stock the carbohydrates, it leads to obesity. Diabetes and cardiovascular disease can result from this cycle. The body behaves more like a fat burner than a carbohydrate-based mechanism. Analysis indicates that a carbohydrate-rich diet is the emergence of a variety of diseases, such as insulin resistance and diabetes.

1.4.1. Diabetes

A ketogenic diet that is known for rich in fats and low in carbohydrates has been found to play a vital role in decreasing and improving specific medical illnesses. It is designated as a part of the cure plan. Carbohydrates are the main source of diabetes. By cutting back on the ingestion in a ketogenic diet, the blood sugar level can be controlled. Other diabetes treatment plans work better in combination with this diet.

1.4.2. Weight Loss

A ketogenic diet has found an obvious position in the conventional dieting trend. It is now part of many fitness or dieting regimen, due to its observed effects of promoting weight loss. Initially, the idea of reducing weight with a rich fat diet upraised many eyebrows and many questions. Over time and as more satisfactory results appeared, a ketogenic diet is now slowly being incorporated as part of weight reduction plans. Carbohydrates lead to gain weight more than fats do. Remember, as we discussed above, that the hormones of insulin help the storage of

carbohydrates so that the weight will be gain. Removing or keeping the carbohydrate consumption to the least can result in considerable weight loss over time.

1.4.3. Cardiovascular Disease

A rich fat diet can be good for health. It depends on the kind and source of fats. Clean and saturated fats in the diet can keep the ingestion of carbohydrates low and improves the body's fat profile. This diet raises the HDL (which is the good cholesterol) levels and takes down the triglyceride levels. This type of fat profile is related to improve the protection against heart strokes and other cardiovascular problems.

1.4.4. Epilepsy

For a certain reason, epileptic attacks are reduced when an individual is on a ketogenic diet. This is the main reason why a ketogenic diet has been introduced. Pediatric epileptic cases are the utmost responsive to this diet. Some kids even have seizure exclusion after a few years of following the ketogenic diet while adult epilepsy has inadequate responses. The children need to fast for a limited day before the beginning of a ketogenic diet plan as a cure for epilepsy.

1.4.5. Cancer

Continuing research shows the potential that a ketogenic diet pushes cancer into reduction. It literally "famishes cancer" to reduce the indications.

1.4.6. Alzheimer's disease

Research illustrates that memory function progresses when a patient with Alzheimer's follows a ketogenic diet. They recover a few of their thought and memory functions.

1.4.7. Neurological disorders

Parkinson's disease and amyotrophic lateral sclerosis (In short ALS) are certain neurological syndromes that benefit from a ketogenic diet. The diet offers mitochondrial support in affected nerves. In this way, the symptoms improve.

1.4.8. Reverse PCOS

One frequently investigated question? Whether keto diet is a good eating technique to help manage PCOS? Different extent of life can be upset due to polycystic ovary syndrome. With other issues, PCOS can also impact weight, and numerous queries come up as to what are the suitable way to cure PCOS via diet. PCOS may be cure with medical treatments such as birth control drugs. But life routine management, such as reducing even a slight weight, might also help lessen the symptoms.

And here's a keto diet question list comes up. That's what needs to know about how a keto can affect PCOS symptoms. The keto diet is a nutritional strategy that emphasizes reducing carbs and taking a high amount of fat so that body uses the fat in energy form. Individuals on the ketogenic diet typically haven't more than 50 grams of carbs per day. As carbs change into glucose in the body, so insulin is required to bring that sugar to the cells to get energy. Like, on the ketogenic diet, the person needs to limit the carb intake, which can assist to relieve the insulin resistance which might occur as an outcome of having PCOS. Also, losing weight and insulin levels can help some women to resume normal ovulation and better fertility.

1.4.9. Efficient against fighting with metabolic syndrome

The possibility of developing diabetes and cardiac failure is typically correlated with metabolic syndrome. Metabolic syndrome contains signs such as:

Abdominal obesity,

High level of blood Pressure

Excessive amounts of sugar in the blood

High level of triglycerides

A low-carbohydrate diet can be successful in maintaining both of these effects, but a keto diet can help hold metabolic syndrome away and can even help reduce weight without bariatric surgery. These symptoms may be removed by adopting the keto diet schedule.

Chapter 2: Menopause and Ketogenic Diet

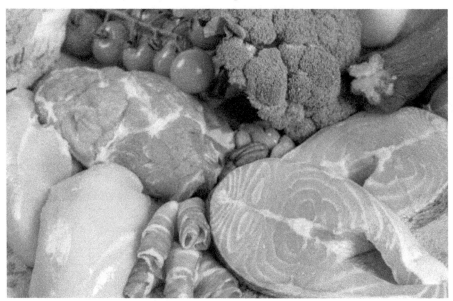

The indicators of menopause can be disturbing for many women. The weight increase, hot flashes, changes in the skin, lack of sleep, low libido, annoyance, and mood fluctuations unsurprisingly happen during this phase. These symptoms can make one feel extremely concerned about the health and well-being. Luckily, we can manage these tough symptoms with healthy habits, starting with the diet. These side effects of menopause are caused by inequities in sex hormones (estrogen and testosterone). A ketogenic diet can help balance these hormones and potentially improve menopause symptoms. In this section, we discuss how we can use a ketogenic diet to manage the symptoms if we're going through menopause.

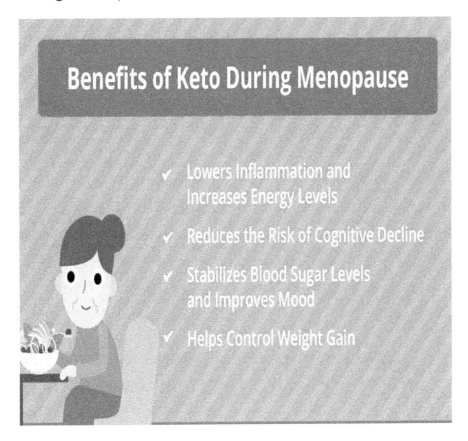

Menopause procedure begins when a woman hasn't had her menstrual period for over twelve months. It usually happens in women over the age of 50 and it is a mark that all of her available eggs have been down. Due to which, estrogen and testosterone, the reproductive hormone level drops. These hormonal changes can generate metabolic difficulties and unwanted symptoms, such as insulin resistance, glucose intolerance, high BP, weight gain, hot flashes, night sweats, loss of libido, and so on so forth. This occurs because all the hormones in the body are linked. Therefore, when the level of reproductive hormones drops, insulin also gets affected, causing metabolic changes. The reduction in testosterone drops the body's ability to build new muscle mass and slowing down the metabolism even more. A reduction in muscle mass and insulin issues leads to fat gain, mainly around your stomach, Inflammation, and oxidative stress, speeding up the aging procedure, encouraging even more weight gain. Auspiciously, adopting a healthy diet that particularly stimulates hormonal balance is one of the coolest ways to improve insulin resistance, maintain muscle mass, lessening inflammation, and maintain a healthy weight. A ketogenic diet, a low carbohydrate, rich in fat diet, has been recognized to diminish a lot of the metabolic issues that happen during menopause because it helps to balance hormones.

2.1. Six ways to improve menopause through keto

A high-fat, low carbohydrate strategy is a ketogenic diet. It's not new, but in recent years, as low-fat, high-carb diets have been seen to be the true culprits behind America's epidemic of obesity, heart disease, and diabetes, it has gained considerable momentum. The new study is being conducted to discover all the possible health benefits, including hormonal factors, with a revived public interest in a ketogenic diet for health and weight loss.

Here are 6 explanations why during menopause a ketogenic diet is beneficial:

1: The Control of Insulin

While no detailed trials have been performed on the complications of keto and menopause, we will learn a lot about the hormonal impact of keto from studies on women with the polycystic ovarian syndrome (PCOS). We've discovered from this analysis that insulin and sex hormones are intricately related. Studies have shown that with a ketogenic diet, normalizing insulin levels can help get sex hormones back into equilibrium, reducing symptoms such as weight gain in women with PCOS. This suggests that you will also regulate sex hormones by raising insulin levels by low carb, high fat diet, and therefore have a decrease in typical menopause symptoms. The influence that keto has on insulin allows it an effective diet to regulate sex hormones and to manage symptoms of menopause.

2: Lose weight

One of the main problems of many women after menopause is weight gain. They may appear to be doing all right, but they are still adding weight The bottom line is that low amounts of estrogen induce weight gain, and it appears to accumulate in the abdominal region in particular. For females who were used to wearing a certain pant size, this may ring warning bells and now nothing matches. They will also continue to cut calories to reduce weight, but this will cause some menopausal symptoms worse. Low-calorie diets delay the metabolism, first of all. They also worsen muscle and bone mass deterioration, increasing the probability of osteoporosis. In itself, menopause often induces muscle and bone deterioration, so why make things worse by consuming a low-calorie diet? The ketogenic diet may be a fantastic way to control weight once you feel the pounds piling up. Evidence suggests that a high-fat diet and low carbs will help women drop weight and hold it off. In a 2015 report, low carbohydrate or low-fat diet was asked to follow postmenopausal women who endured breast cancer. In six months, those who adopted the low-carb diet dropped 23.1 pounds, 7.6 percent body weight, and 3.7 inches in their waist. Although both groups lost weight, substantially more was lost by the low carb group. There are many explanations that a keto diet leads to weight management and can make it easier for women during menopause to sustain a healthier weight. Larger consumption of protein improves satiety. You're less inclined to overeat when you feel complete and satisfied. In comparison, the reduction of most carbohydrates also results in reduced calorie consumption overall. A ketogenic diet regulates the chemicals of starvation. A 2013 research discovered that participants had healthy amounts of ghrelin after 8 weeks on a ketogenic diet. In certain carb-based diets, ghrelin is an appetite-stimulating hormone that enhances desire. Subjects have lost 13% of their body weight in the same sample and had lower overall hunger ratings. Keto accelerates digestion and the burning of calories. Several calories are absorbed by gluconeogenesis, or by the processing of glucose from non-carb compounds. Metabolism is often accelerated by lipolysis or the breakdown of fat for energy. Any diet that speeds up the metabolism would be helpful for women who suffer a metabolic slowdown. The bottom line is that some of the weight gain encountered in menopause can help stave off the ketogenic diet and may help normalize metabolism.

3: Hot Flashes Elimination

Hot flashes are an exceedingly annoying menopause complication. They will interrupt your sleep and make you feel very unpleasant. While the precise cause of hot flashes is not understood, low estrogen levels and their influence on the hypothalamus is presumably linked to them, a part of the brain that controls body temperature. Ketone bodies formed during ketosis can help protect the brain and minimize inflammation, which can help to control the temperature of the body.

4: Regulation between Sex Hormones

Because of such fluctuating hormones, lack of libido can be one side effect of menopause. A high-fat diet will, therefore, serve to boost both the levels of estrogen and testosterone, contributing to raising libido. Sex hormones are manufactured from fat. It was seen to decrease circulating sex hormones after a low-fat diet and may in turn decrease libido. Research has also shown the reverse, that in women, consuming a higher fat diet increases sexual function. Consuming a high-fat, ketogenic diet provides the body the raw materials it requires to sustain quantities of sex hormones, an essential component in sustaining a stable menopausal libido

5: High energy levels

In terms of energy levels, ketogenic diets may also help. There are no longer big swings of blood sugar that induce energy declines as the body switches to using fat for energy instead of carbohydrates. Your body also now has an almost infinite supply of calories (your fat stores) to tap into, growing the energy levels anytime it wants to.

6: Great Sleep, Better Sleep

During menopause, following a ketogenic diet will even boost sleep. Healthy sleep would be a great symptom, due to the elimination of hot flashes, better blood sugar control, healthier weight, and hormone balance. It's time to put it into effect now that you know how a ketogenic diet will better relieve the effects of menopause and boost your general wellbeing.

Chapter 3: Do's and Don'ts of Ketogenic Diet

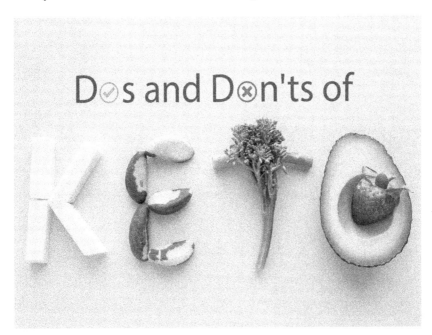

Among individuals with health & wellness aspirations, weight reduction, blood glucose regulation, and increased athletic efficiency, a ketogenic diet has become a common alternative. You might make errors that keep you from completing ketosis if you're new to the diet.

We're going to teach you in this book how to successfully execute the diet with our collection of dos and don'ts. To keep on track, you may also want this list. Continue to learn.

3.1. Do's of Keto diet

1. Prepare the food list for a ketogenic diet.

What should I consume with this keto diet? "If you ever catch yourself posing this question, reading a collection of ketogenic approved recipes would aid. Keep for diets that are rich in fat and low carbohydrates. Fatty meat pieces, plants, eggs & dairy are examples. Keep your products and preparations basic, since it requires time to adapt to the diet. You shouldn't be scared to try as long as we satisfy the micronutrient & macronutrient requirements.

2. Take a full meal.

It is a fact that there are a lot of processed snacks that make them easy to consume. Packaged drugs, though, can include poor fats and sugars that come with different labels, such as Agave Nectar, Maltodextrin, Dextran, and more. The way to maintain optimal quality is by consuming foods in their usual state. Whole foods, which help avoid micronutrient malnutrition, are abundant in minerals & vitamins. Choose minimally processed foods instead, if you're particularly busy.

3. Eat lots of healthy fat.

This mistake is made by several keto dieters; they consume extra fat but do not pay heed to the quality of the fats. Although having 60-75 percent of the calories from the fats is essential, you have to make it clear that calories come from polyunsaturated fats & good monounsaturated and Note that there is typically a healthy form of fat present in seafood, nuts, beans, and vegetables. Sardines, walnuts, Salmon, pecans, lettuce, flaxseed, and avocados are several examples.

4. Check the levels of blood glucose.

Keto aims to bring the body into a condition of ketosis. You should maintain the glucose of blood under control (approx. less than 100 mg/dL) for you to do it.

Watching for fluctuations in the sugar levels when you're doing keto makes sense. This is particularly valid if you attempt alternative "keto" diets, encounter tension, or evaluate the efficacy of fasting. It is therefore recommended for patients with type 2 diabetes to observe the blood glucose periodically.

5. Lookout for sugars that are concealed.

Done all the prescribed by the keto routine, but don't see results Maybe you deal with an adversary, secret carbohydrates. It doesn't mean that you're in ketosis simply because you're skipping rice, noodles, and pastries.

Several fat-free dressings appear to be full of sugar. Coleslaw, Greek yogurt, Sauces, condiments, and cashew nuts are certain types of secret carbohydrates. Amazed? To prevent these secret carbohydrates, the easiest option is to prepare your food in your home.

6. Always drink plenty of fluid like water.

Ketosis is considered to cause multiple side effects. Dehydration is one of these adverse effects. Some persons urinate more often than have ketosis. This arises because glycogen stocks are decreasing in their bodies. If you don't know what actually glycogen is, it's the primary source of glucose storage. You need to improve your water consumption on keto. It would also help to stop stones in the kidney and relieve headaches by doing so. Try adding any berries, ice, or cucumbers into the water to meet the water consumption targets.

7. Take supplements containing vitamins and minerals.

On keto, should you take supplements of vitamins and minerals? The response is "indeed yes". Because you cut off several ingredients, a ketogenic diet will cause deficiencies of minerals and vitamins. Some individuals often do not adopt a well-balanced keto diet by consuming something fatty, especially bad fat. Poor fats sometimes lack nutrients. Ensure that you receive sufficiently zinc, B-complex, vitamin D, magnesium, sodium, vitamin C, and vitamins. Apart from a multivitamin supplement, select whole food.

8. Be prepare for keto flu

There's a set of symptoms that certain individuals who initiate keto encounter. These effects are recognized as "keto flu." As the body removes from carbs, keto flu arises. Headaches, dizziness, nausea, stomach cramps, and muscle weakening are the recorded signs.

Always note that people respond differently to keto. Some have and some don't have the keto flu. However, one needs to follow to reduce these symptoms: stop strenuous exercise, get enough sleep, drink sufficient water, raise good fat consumption, and substitute electrolytes.

3.2. Don'ts of Keto Diet

1. Eat food that is low in fat. Since keto is a rich-fat diet, prioritizing items that contain more fat makes sense. Research has also found that the sugar level in less-calorie items such as baked goods and dairy products is greater. It doesn't mean that they are low-sugar simply because the labels claim less-calorie." Your ketogenic diet provides multiple options to incorporate more fat. You should add cheese to your meals that are made up of vegetables. Make recipes of avocado, drizzle salads with olive oil, and use MCT oil.

2. Use underground-grown veggies.

Keto is perfect for cruciferous vegetables and those veggies which grown up on the ground. These vegetables have less sugar and are full of antioxidants and nutrients. Cauliflower, cabbage, broccoli, and spinach are low-carb choices. Onions, sweet potatoes, beets maize, peas can be prohibited.

3. Chewing so many nuts

Always remember that all nuts are equally made. As somebody on keto, for your choices and quantity of nuts, you must be cautious. Cashews, pistachios, and pine have nuts that appear to contain lots of carbs. Pecans, Brazil and macadamias, are the types of keto nuts. Always remember that while rich-carb and low-carb nuts are present, you should not go overboard with nuts in particular. It's nice to eat nuts, but when you need energy, not when you're hungry and just need anything to chew on.

4. Using the keto diet for a fast cure.

A keto diet is not an immediate effective diet. It's a mode of life, a lifestyle. We see so many individuals getting in this diet to easily lose weight and they stop immediately if they don't. Any persons, when they get keto flu, feel frustrated due to lack of study. Another myth is that ketogenic diet and low-carb are similar things. Having a better understanding of what ketosis is? Is it the easiest way to tackle keto? Know your research, your accurate macros of keto, and expect any improvements.

5. Without referring to the doctor, pursue Keto.

It will be nice to speak up about your keto diet if you see a specialist or you have a health problem (for instance, diabetes or any heart disease). Since there could be drugs that contraindicate keto, the doctor needs to know your dietetic strategy. Most notably, inform your doctor about your keto encounter. Have you gained more energy? Has the blood glucose reduced?

Hopefully, these do's and don'ts can boost the adhesion to a ketogenic diet. Choose more genuine ingredients and healthy fats to bring out the best results from the diet. Don't ignore the requirements for micronutrients. As a diet, accept keto, instead of an instant cure. Keep yourself updated.

3.3. Restricted food

To cause ketosis, carbohydrates are primarily limited. The body, however, will adjust to dietary change. Proteins, thus, and Fats, too, ought to be monitored.

- Fats

  In a ketogenic diet, fats are usually promoted. It is the predominant source of energy during ketosis. Approximately 60% to 80% of total calories are supposed to come with fats. The value depends on a ketogenic diet's target. Some can also use fats as 90% of the overall dietary intake.

  However, when deciding the kind of fats to use, there are a few rules to consider. No omega-6 polyunsaturated fats. Insignificant concentrations, omega-6 fats appear to be inflammatory.

- Corn oil

- Soy

- Cottonseed

 Stop seed or nut-based oils since they are rich in omega-6 and may hurt the body.

- Almond oil

- Flaxseeds

- Sesame Seed Oil

- Stop mayonnaise and dressings with commercial salads. If inevitable, verify the carbohydrate material.

- Stop fats and Trans fats that are hydrogenated.

These were found to be correlated with increased risk for the production of coronary heart issues and other health complications.

- The Proteins

It is critical to select proteins since they will influence the diet over time. Steroid-treated and antibiotic-treated animals can cause problems with health. Choose grass-fed, free-range, and natural. Ignore those who have been fed with hormones, particularly RBST.

However, review the starch content that could come from the use of extenders or fillers while selecting processed meat items. Avoid any curing meat that contains honey or sugar.

- Carbohydrates

In specific, ketogenic diets impose extreme limits on the consumption of carbohydrates. The restriction is based on the level of activity of the person and level of metabolism. Generally, a net daily carbohydrate consumption of less than 50 or 60 grams is needed for a ketogenic diet. Individuals with healthy metabolism (such as athletes) can intake as many as 100 or more grams per day. It could be important for sedentary individuals with type 2 diabetes mellitus to limit carbohydrates to less than 30 grams in a day. It relies on tolerance and the state of wellbeing. The aim of a keto diet is also based on it.

- Vegetables

Although the key sources of carbohydrates in a ketogenic diet are vegetables, some need to be prevented. Some veggies have large amounts of sugar such as peppers, tomatoes, and onions. The bulk of vegetables that grow underground are starchy, producing plenty of starch.

- The Sweets

The typical sweet foods are completely avoided since they are very rich in sugars and carbohydrates. They are:

- Cakes

- Sweetbread

- Bread and buns

- Glace-fruit

- Chocolates: These contain diet chocolate and other types of chocolate, including lollipops. Biscuits: normal, iced, or chocolate-coated, with cream filling

- Pies

- Pastry

- Puddings

- Sweetened toppings and syrups

- Milk condensed

- Ice-creams

- Jam: all kinds, such as diabetic jam

- Milk flavorings

- Drinks such as Ovaltine, Milo

- Sauces

- Chutneys and pickles

- Flavored yogurt- Artificial flavoring may include sugar as malt dextrin or in any other shape.

- Cordials and sugar-containing soft beverages.

- Fruit Juice

- Chewing gum, including some who are sugarless

- Sweetened syrups and treatments for coughing

- Sugars

    Sugar is a rich carbohydrate supply that needs to be stopped. Sugar is commonly known in ways such as brown sugar, white sugar, castor, and icing. In refined foods and medicines, it may also be an element

3.4. Permitted Food

In a ketogenic diet, meals consist predominantly of 3 specific forms of food. There's a fruit, a diet high in proteins, and a source of fat.

- Fats

    The ketogenic diet calls for extra fatty fats. They may be used, such as frying or pan grilling, as part of the cooking method. Fats may also be in the form of sauces and dressings. A way of adding fats into the diet is often to simply top a slice of steak with butter. Those that are ketogenic are the better form of fat.

The MCTs or medium-chain triglycerides are the best, which involve MCT oil and coconut oil. To generate ketones, these fats are readily metabolized.

For ketosis, other healthy fats are:

- Omega-3 and Omega-6 Fatty acids

- Trout

- Salmon

- Tuna

- Shellfish

- Saturated and monounsaturated fats

- Olive oil

- Red palm-oil

- Butter

- Cheese

- Avocado

- Egg yolks

- Non-hydrogenated oil (when cooking)

- Tallow beef

- Lards that are non-hydrogenated

- Coconut oil

- High oleic acid

- Oils of Safflower

- Sunflowers oil

- Peanut-butter

- Skin of chicken

- Fat of beef

- Coconut butter

- The Proteins

In a keto diet, every form of meat is effectively permitted. The sort of cut or preparation should not differentiate.

- Pork
- Beef
- Veal
- Venison
- Lamb
- Poultry

Use every sort of poultry item. It is preferable to have the skin on since it improves the meal's fat quality. As they have high carbohydrate content, preparation does not require the use of breading and batter. Acceptable preparations are based on an individual's choice.

- Chicken
- Quail

- Turkey
- Duck
- Sea Foods

Seafood is a decent source of protein as well. Some include elevated amounts of omega-3 fatty acids, vitamins, and minerals that can help sustain proper nutrition for healthier people.

Fish has a large content of safe omega-3 fatty acids. Choose fish that are captured in the wild and places clear of mercury.

- Tuna
- Catfish
- Halibut
- Flounder
- Cod
- Snapper
- Trout
- Salmon
- Mackerel
- Shellfish
- Clams
- Squid
- Mahi-mahi
- Oysters
- Lobster
- Mussel
- Scallops
- Carbohydrates

- Vegetables

The primary sources of carbohydrates in a ketogenic diet involve vegetables. There are excellent opportunities for organically raised vegetables. There isn't much difference between organic and non-organic in terms of nutritional value. The difference lies in the risk of eating vegetables treated with dark leafy vegetables with the lowest nutritionally valuable carbohydrate content.

- Spinach
- Watercress
- Cabbage, all sorts
- Lettuce, both forms
- Kale
- Sprouts from Brussels
- Broccoli
- Celery
- Cucumber
- Cauliflower
- Bean sprout
- Radishes
- Asparagus
- Dairy and Milk Goods

In a ketogenic diet, milk and dairy items are fundamental. There is a preference for natural and renewable sources. It is often easier to select the complete fat varieties than the fat-free or reduced-fat versions. In a ketogenic diet, eggs are staples

It is a perfect source of fats and proteins.

Cheese, from hard to soft kinds. There are carbs in it. Include the cheeses in the daily carbohydrates count. Some of them are:

- Mascarpone
- Cheddar
- Mozzarella
- Cream cheese
- Cottage cheese

It is therefore advised that sour cream be used in the diet. It serves more interesting varieties.

- Nuts

In a ketogenic diet, a reasonable intake of nuts is permitted. Proteins, fats, and carbohydrates are rich in them. The Variety of Nuts needs to be observed for carbohydrate, fats, and protein ingredients and included in the regular keto estimation.

Roasted nuts and Seeds are the safest since they eliminate something in the body that may inflict damage or mess with ketosis. Nuts are mainly promoted as a snack. Almonds, macadamias, and walnuts are the right nuts for inclusion. Some nuts are high in omega-6 fatty acids, which in the body can induce inflammation. Pistachio and cashew produce higher carbohydrate levels. Best to slowly rack these up.

- Spices

It may be tough to adapt to fewer carbohydrate consumption within the first several weeks after adopting a ketogenic diet. Individuals who have the sweet tooth can find it too hard to handle in their cravings. People that are used to consuming meals of high carbohydrates such as spaghetti and pasta or processed foods can complain of boring meals that are less tasty. After some time, ketogenic foods will become boring. Spices can spice things up. You may add fresh and dried spices to the meals and also beverages to make the meals a little more tempting and entertaining. Spices have carbohydrates. Few spices should include in daily carbs and ketogenic count. Typically, pre-made spice mixes include added sugar. To add the accurate amount of total carbohydrates, count, one should read the labels of the content

This is the form of sugar that should be avoided in a ketogenic diet. Not just for the tastes, but also for the different health benefits that they bring, spices may be included. Some of these advantageous spices Includes:

- Basil
- Black pepper
- Cayenne pepper
- Cilantro
- Cinnamon
- Dust of chili
- Cumin
- Parsley

- Oregano
- Sage
- Rosemary
- Turmeric
- Thyme
- Sweeteners

In curbing cravings for food and sweets, artificial sweeteners are beneficial. They lead to achieving progress in adhering to a Ketogenic diet. Using chemical sweeteners such as Stevia and E-Z Sweets is safest. Carbohydrate count does not impact them. When sweeteners, since no binders such as dextrose and maltodextrin have been

added, the liquid form is preferred.

Some of the suggested sweeteners are listed below:

- Sucralose (the liquid form is recommended)
- Xylitol
- Erythritol
- Monk fruits
- The Beverages

The low ingestion of carbohydrates in the body has a diuretic impact. Carbohydrates draw water into them, leading to the retention of water by lowering the carbohydrates in the diet, a very little amount of water is retained and more is excreted.

This may render a person predisposed to dehydration. It is a necessity to consume sufficient volumes of water daily. The likelihood of diseases of the urinary tract and bladder discomfort often rises as the body is losing more water.

The low ingestion of carbohydrates in the body has a diuretic impact. Carbohydrates draw water into them, leading to the retention of water. By lowering the carbohydrates in the diet, a very little amount of water is retained and more is excreted. This may render a person predisposed to dehydration. It is a necessity to consume sufficient volumes of water daily. The likelihood of diseases of the urinary tract and bladder discomfort often rises as the body is losing more water.

Drink more than the normal regular consumption of 8 glasses of water suggested. To increase, the hydration status, add other forms of beverages. Coffee and tea can also be added to daily liquid intake. Only coffee and tea do not affect the ketosis but the added ingredients into it will work for sure. Choose artificial sweeteners. Whether, drink full-cream coffee or tea and omit all the sugar together. Instead of fruit smoothies, power smoothies or protein shakes are better to use. Sugars that may inhibit ketosis are found in the fruits.

- Vegetable juice

When on a ketogenic diet, using the permitted vegetable forms is also great to drink ideas.

Chapter 4: Keto Meal Plan

Planning is important for progress on a ketogenic diet. This chapter of the book will show you how to make a meal idea for a ketogenic diet to fit your needs and objectives.

We have broken it down into five stages to help you build the right meal idea for yourself.

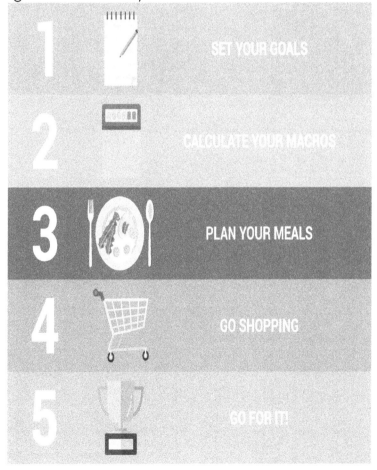

1. Set the goal

What is the purpose of consuming a ketogenic diet for you? Think of the outcomes you'd like to achieve, whether it's weight reduction, improved emotional clarity, avoidance of illness, or better physical wellbeing. Write them down somewhere the day you see them. It would help to adapt your meal plans to your needs with this in mind beforehand, as well as making it easy to adhere to your keto diet.

2. Evaluate the macros

On a ketogenic diet, macronutrient levels are very important. On a ketogenic diet, consider the macro ratios. Based on your body composition and lifestyle,

working from here will allow you to decide whether and how much of each category to consume.

3. Plan the meal

Planning what you'll consume depends on your regular macros! You could be preparing for a few days or at a time for the entire week. Most keto recipes have a list macro breakdown so you don't have to quantify it. You can check ingredients to a diet app if they don't, for their macros and calorie count.

Decide which meals each day you'll get. On a sheet of paper, it helps to list them out. Consider that:

How many people can eat the meals in your home (or how many servings you'll need to make)

How you like each day to be planned. Do you intend on having breakfast, for instance, or are you already going to have lunch and dinner most days?

When your meals are set, make a grocery list for each meal with the items you'll need. The ingredients are grouped by types, such as "meat," "dairy," "vegetables," etc.

Time to go to the grocery now!

4. Go on a shopping

A simple rule of thumb: buy first the perimeter of the store. That's where they place fresh fruit, poultry, and milk goods.

The internal aisles for oils and other specific keto stuff will need to be visited, but shopping on the outside first eliminates overwhelm, lets you concentrate on the healthiest items, and makes it easier to avoid some junky processed stuff that is surely not keto-friendly (out of sight, out of mind).

5. Go for it,

Your ingredients are yours. You've planned the meals Perhaps most of your meals ought to be

made and cooked ahead of time and stored for quik grab 'N go.

4.2. Keto Diet grocery list

Here we list out those items which should be needed to start the keto process.

4.2.1 List of Week 1

Meat

- Thick-cut pork, 24 strips

- Beef, ground (80% lean)-30 ounces

- Thighs of chicken, boneless-2 pounds

- Eggs-17 large-sized

- Ham, delicatessen, sliced-3 ounces

- Ham, 6 ounces' fat-free

- Salmon, boneless-4 fillets (6-ounce)

Vegetables and Fruits

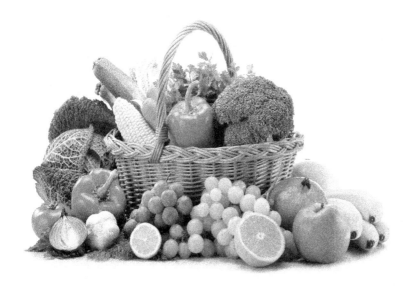

- 1 bunch of asparagus

- Avocado- 3 thin, 3 medium-sized

- Beets: 1 tiny beet

- Bell pepper, red—1 small, 1 small

- Cauliflower- 2 cups

- Chives- 1 bunch of chives

- Cucumber, English-Medium 1 1/2

- Garlic- 1 head

- Kale: 1 cup

- Lemon-1

- 5 cups of lettuce

- Mushrooms-1 cup

- Onion, red—1 tiny, 1 small

- Onion, yellow—1 short, 1 medium

- Spinach - 2 cups

- Tomatoes -1/2 cup of tomatoes

- Zucchini: 1 tiny, 1 wide

Frozen and Refrigerated Products

- Unsweetened almond milk- 1 3/4 cups

- Blueberries, 1/4 cup frozen

- Cheddar cheese, shredded-1 3/4 cups

- Unsweetened coconut milk, 1 cup

- 9 ounces' cream cheese

- Strong cream-1/4 cup

- Mayonnaise- 3 teaspoons of mayonnaise

- Parmesan ham rubbed—1 cup

- Provolone cheese, 1/4 cup shredded

- Sour cream: 1 cup

- Yogurt, full-fat-3/4 cup

Staples and Dry Products Pantry

- Almonds, whole, 1 cup

- 1 cup plus 1 tablespoon of almond butter

- 1/2 cup almond flour

- Vinegar with apple cider

- Basil pesto-1/4 cup

- Black pepper

- Soup, beef, 3 cups

- Chia seeds—1 teaspoon

- Powder of Chili

- Powder of chocolate, unsweetened

- 1/4 cup coconut flour

- Coconut Oil

- Tartar milk

- Mustard from Dijon

- Ground cinnamon •

- Ground Cumin •

- Olive Oil

- Liquid extract of stevia

- 16 macadamia nuts

- Paprika

- Erythritol dried

- Protein powder, white egg, vanilla-1/4 cup

- Pumpkin bread cinnamon spice

- Seasoning ranch

- Salt

- Tomato paste- 2 teaspoons of the paste

4.2.2 List of Week 2

Meat

- Thick-cut pork, 19 strips

- Thighs of chicken, boneless-2 pounds

- Eggs - 26 large eggs

- Ham, delicatessen, diced-1/4 cup

- Ham, free of fat: 2 pounds plus 1 ounce

- Tenderloin of bacon, boneless-1 1/2 pounds

- Salmon, boneless - 8 ounces

- Tuna, ahi-4 steaks (6-ounce)

Vegetables and Fruits

- Avocado- 2 short, 2 medium

- Green bell pepper, 1 tiny

- Cauliflower: three cups

- Celery- 1 tiny stalk

- Garlic- 1 head

- 1 bit of ginger

- Green beans, 2 cups

- Lemon-1

- Lettuce-4 1/4 cups

- Onion, red—1 tiny, 1 small

- Onion, purple, 1 tiny

- 1 bunch of parsley

- Rosemary-one bunch

- 4 ounces spring greens

- Tomato- 1 tiny tomato

Frozen and Refrigerated Products

- Almond oil, an unsweetened-3/4 cup of milk

- Butter - 1 tablespoon of butter

- Cream cheese, 1 ounce

- 1 cup plus 1 tablespoon heavy cream

- Mayonnaise- 3 teaspoons of mayonnaise

- Parmesan, 1/4 cup shaved

- Staples and Dry Products Pantry

- Almond butter: 1 3/4 cups

- 2 1/2 cups almond flour

- Baking Powder

- Black pepper

- Broth, chicken-five cups

- 1/2 cup of Chia seeds

- Bouillon of chicken-4 cubes

- Paste with chili garlic

- Powder of chocolate, unsweetened

- 2 teaspoons of coconut flour

- Coconut oil, canned-3 1/4 cups

- Coconut Oil

- Tartar milk

- Dijon Mustard

- 2 scoops of egg white protein powder (40g)

- Garam masala

- Ground cinnamon

- Ground Nutmeg

- Guar gum

- Olive Oil

- Powder of Onion

- Liquid extract of stevia

- Pine nuts, 1/3 cup roasted

- Erythritol dried

- Vinegar from red wine

- Salt

- Sesame beans, black-1⁄4 cup

- Sesame beans, toasted-1⁄2 cup

- Sesame beans, white-1⁄4 cup

- Smoked paprika

- 3 tbsp. tomato paste

- Extract of vanilla

- Sesame oil

- Soy sauce

- Extract of vanilla

4.3. Keto Diet Pyramid

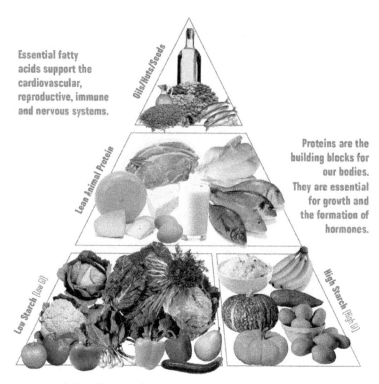

Essential fatty acids support the cardiovascular, reproductive, immune and nervous systems.

Oils/Nuts/Seeds

Lean Animal Protein

Proteins are the building blocks for our bodies. They are essential for growth and the formation of hormones.

Low Starch (Low GI)

High Starch (High GI)

Carbohydrates are broken down in the body to give us energy.

Chapter 5: Ketogenic diet meal recipes.

5.1. Recipes for breakfast

1. Veggies and Parmesan with Sheet Pan Eggs

Servings: 6 Servings:

Prep Time: 5 minutes

Cooking time: 15 minutes

Ingredients:

- 12 big, whisked eggs

- Salt and pepper

- 1 tiny red pepper, diced

- 1 tiny yellow, chopped onion

- 1 cup of diced mushrooms

- 1 cup of zucchini diced

- 1 cup of Parmesan cheese freshly grated

Instructions:

1. Preheat the oven to 350 ° F and then grease a rimmed baking sheet with cooking spray.

2. In a cup, whisk the eggs until frothy with salt and pepper.

3. Stir in the tomatoes, mushrooms, onions, and zucchini until well combined.

4. In the baking pan, pour the mixture and scatter it into an even layer.

5. Sprinkle with parmesan and bake until the egg is set, for 12 to 15 minutes.

6. Let it cool slowly, then slice it into serving squares.

Nutrition Info: 215 calories, 14g of fat, 18.5g of protein, 5g of carbohydrates, 1g of fiber, 4g of net carbohydrates.

2. Tomato Mozzarella Egg Muffins
Servings: 12 Servings:

Time to prep: 5 minutes

Cook Time: Twenty-five minutes

Ingredients:

- 1 tablespoon of butter

- 1 tomato medium, finely diced

- 1/2 cup of yellow onion diced

- 12 big, whisked eggs

- 1/2 cup of coconut milk canned

- 1/4 cup of green onion cut

- Salt and pepper

- 1 cup of mozzarella cheese shredded

Instructions:

1. Preheat the oven to 350 ° F and grease the pan with cooking spray.

2. In a medium skillet over medium heat, melt the butter.

3. Put the tomatoes and onions in the pan and cook until tender, for 3 to 4 minutes.

4. Pour the mixture into muffin cups.

5. Combine the eggs, coconut milk, green onions, salt, and pepper, and mix properly. Then put a spoon in the muffin cup.

6. Sprinkle with cheese, then bake until the egg is set, for 20 to 25 minutes.

Nutrition Information: 135 calories, 10.5g of fat, 9g of protein, 2g of carbohydrates, 0.5g of fiber, 1.5g of carbohydrates.

3. Cinnamon & Almond Porridge
Servings: 1 Serving:

Prep time: 5 minutes

Cook time: 5 minutes

Ingredients:

- 1 tablespoon of butter

- 1 tablespoon of coconut flour

- 1 large egg, whisked

- 1/8 teaspoon cinnamon powder

- Pinch of salt

- 1/4 cup of canned coconut milk

- 1 almond butter tablespoon

Instructions:

1. In a medium saucepan over a low flame, melt the butter.

2. Put the coconut flour, egg, cinnamon, and salt and whisk.

3. While whisking, add the coconut milk and stir in the almond butter until well smooth.

4. Simmer over low heat, stirring regularly, until fully heated.

5. Spoon and serve in a bowl.

Nutrition Information: 470 calories, 42g of fat, 13g of protein, 15g of carbohydrates, 8g of fiber, 7g of net carbohydrates

4. Crispy Chai Waffles
Servings: 4 Servings:

Prep time: 10 minutes

Cook time: 20 minutes

Ingredients:

- Four large eggs separated into whites and yolks

- 3 teaspoons of coconut flour

- 3 teaspoons erythritol powder

- 1 1/4 teaspoon baking powder

- 1 teaspoon Vanilla extract

- 1/2 teaspoon ground cinnamon

- 1/4 teaspoon of ground ginger

- Ground cloves pinch

- Cardamom ground pinch

- 3 teaspoons of molten coconut oil

- 3 teaspoons almond milk unsweetened

Instructions:

1. Separate the eggs into two separate bowls.

2. Whip the egg whites until they stiff peaks and put aside.

3. Whisk the coconut flour with the egg yolks, erythritol, baking powder,

add vanilla, cinnamon, cardamom, and cloves in another bowl.

4. When whisking, apply the molten coconut oil to the second bowl and whisk

in almond milk.

5. Fold the egg whites carefully until they're combined.

6. Grease the preheated waffle iron with cooking spray.

7. Spoon 1/2 cup or so of batter onto the iron.

8. Cook the waffle according to directions from the maker.

9. Remove the waffle to a plate and repeat with the batter that remains.

Nutrition Information: 215 calories, 17g of fat, 8g of protein, 8g of carbohydrates,

4g of fiber, 4g of net weight,

5. Sheet Pan Eggs with Ham and Pepper Jack
Servings: 6 Servings:

Time to prep: 5 minutes

Cook time: 15 minutes

Ingredients:

- 12 big, whisked eggs

- Salt and pepper

- Two cups of sliced ham

- 1 cup of shredded cheese and pepper jack

Instructions:

1. Preheat the oven to 350 ° F and cook a rimmed baking sheet with oil.

2. In a cup, whisk the eggs until frothy with salt and pepper.

3. Stir in the cheese and ham once well mixed.

4. In the baking pan, pour the mixture and scatter it into an even layer.

5. Bake until the egg is set, for 12 to 15 minutes.

6. Then leave to cool slightly and cut into squares to eat.

Nutrition information: 235 calories, 15g of fat, 21g of protein, 2.5g of carbohydrates, 0.5g of fiber, 2g of net carbohydrates.

5.2 Recipes for lunch

1. Three Meat & Cheese Sandwich
Servings: 1 Serving

Prep Time: 30 minutes

Cook time: 5 minutes

Ingredients:

- 2 big eggs,

- 1 pinch cream of tartar

- Pinch of salt

- 1 ounce of softened cream cheese

- 1 ounce of ham cut

- 1 ounce of hard salami cut

- 1 ounce of turkey cut

- 2 cheddar cheese slices

Instructions:

1. Preheat the oven to 300 °F for the bread and line a baking sheet with

Parchment.

2. Beat the egg whites with tartar cream and salt until it becomes soft peaks.

3. Whisk the egg yolk and cream cheese until smooth and pale yellow.

4. Gradually mix the yolk batter into the egg whites until smooth and well mixed.

5. Pour the mixture into two even circles onto the baking dish.

6. Bake until solid and slightly browned, for 25 minutes.

7. Make a sandwich by putting the sliced meat and cheese between two bread slices.

8. With cooking oil, grease a skillet and heat over low flame.

9. Keep the sandwich on the skillet and cook until the bottom has browned, then flip and cook until the cheese melts.

Nutrition Information: 610 calories, 48g of fat, 40g of protein, 3g of carbohydrates,

0.5g of fiber, 2.5g of carbohydrates

2. Kebabs of Beef and Pepper
Servings: 2 Servings

Prep time: 30 minutes

Cook time: 10 minutes

Ingredients:

- 2 teaspoons of olive oil

- 1 1/2 teaspoons of balsamic vinegar

- 2 teaspoons of Dijon mustard

- Salt and pepper

- Beef sirloin, 8 ounces, sliced into 2-inch pieces

- 1 tiny red pepper, chopped into pieces

- 1 tiny green pepper, chopped into pieces

Instructions:

1. In a small dish, mix the olive oil, balsamic vinegar, and Dijon mustard.

2. Season the steak with salt and pepper and then toss in the marinade.

3. Let it marinate for 30 minutes, then slide it with peppers onto skewers.

4. Preheat the grill pan to high flame and use the cooking spray to grease.

5. Cook the kebabs on either side for 2 to 3 minutes until the beef is cooked.

Nutrition Information: 365 calories, 21.5g of fat, 35.5g of protein, 6.5g of carbohydrates, 1.5g of fiber, 5g of net carbohydrates

3. Chicken tenders with Coconut
Servings: 4 Servings

Prep time: 10 minutes

Cook time: 30 minutes

Ingredients:

- 1/4 cup of almond flour

- 2 teaspoons of unsweetened shredded coconut

- 1/2 tablespoons of garlic powder

- 2 pounds of boneless chicken

- Salt and pepper

- 2 big eggs, well whisked,

Instructions:

1. Preheat the oven to 400 ° F and use parchment to cover a baking sheet.

2. In a small bowl, mix the almond flour, coconut, and garlic powder.

3. Season the chicken with salt and pepper, then dip in the beaten eggs.

4. In the almond flour mixture, dredge the chicken tenders, then place them on

the baking sheet.

5. Bake for 25 to 30 minutes, until baked and browned. Serve it hot.

Nutrition Facts: 325 calories, 9.5g of fat, 56.5g of protein, 2g of carbohydrates, 1g

of fiber, 1g net carbohydrates.

4. Ham, Egg & Cheese Sandwich
Servings: 1 Serving:

Prep time: 30 minutes

Cook time: 5 minutes

Ingredients:

- 2 big eggs

- Tartar pinch milk

- Pinch of salt

- 1 ounce of cream cheese, melted

- 1 butter teaspoon

- 3 ounces of ham cut

- 1 cheddar cheese slice

Instructions

1. Preheat the oven to 300 °F for the bread and line a baking sheet with

Parchment.

2. Beat the egg whites with tartar cream and salt until becomes soft peaks.

3. Whisk the egg yolk and cream cheese until smooth and pale yellow.

4. Mix the egg yolk batter into egg whites until smooth and well mixed.

5. Pour the batter into two even circles onto the baking dish.

6. Bake approx. for 25 minutes until it becomes firm and slightly brown.

7. Fry the egg in butter until it's done as per your requirement.

8. On top of one bread circle, place the sliced ham.

9. Cover that with the sliced cheese and the fried egg, then the second circle of bread.

10. Serve immediately or toast it until cheese is melt.

Nutrition information: 530 calories, 40g of fat, 36g of protein, 5.5g of

carbohydrates, 1g of fiber, 4.5g of total carbohydrates.

5.Curried Chicken Soup
Servings: 4 Servings:

Prep time: 10 minutes

Cook time: 20 minutes

Ingredients:

- 2 teaspoons of olive oil

- 4 thighs of boneless chicken (about 12 ounces)

- 1 tiny yellow, chopped onion

- 2 teaspoons of curry powder

- 2 teaspoons of cumin seed powder

- Pinch of cayenne

- 4 cups of cauliflower

- 4 cups of chicken broth

- 1 cup of water

- 2 minced garlic cloves

- 1/2 cup of canned coconut milk

- 2 cups of chopped kale

- Freshly chopped cilantro

Instructions:

1. Chop the chicken into bite-sized pieces and put it aside.

2. Over medium flame, heat 1 tablespoon of oil in a saucepan.

3. Sauté the onions for 4 minutes, then add half the spices to it.

4. Add the cauliflower and sauté further four minutes.

5. Add water and garlic to the broth and boil it.

6. Low the flame and cook for 10 minutes until the cauliflower softens.

7. Remove from the heat and add kale and coconut milk.

8. In a pan, heat the remaining oil and cook the chicken until it turns golden brown.

9. Stir in the remaining spices and cook until the chicken has been done.

10. Mix the chicken with broth and serve it hot, garnished with fresh cilantro.

Nutrition Information: 390 calories, 22 g fat, 34 g protein, 14.5 g carbohydrates,

4.5g fiber, 10 g net carbohydrates.

5.3. Recipes for dinner

1.   Baked Lamb Chops with Asparagus
Servings: 4 Servings

Time to prep: 5 minutes

Cook time: 15 minutes

Ingredients:

- 8 bone-in chops of lamb

- Salt and pepper

- 1 tablespoon freshly chopped rosemary

- 1 tablespoon of olive oil

- 1 tablespoon of butter

- 16 asparagus spears, sliced into 2-inch chunks

Instructions:

1. Season the salt and pepper with the lamb and sprinkle the rosemary.

2. Heat oil over medium-high flame in a large skillet.

3. Put the lamb chops and cook until seared, on both sides, for 2 to 3 minutes.

1.   Remove the chops from the skillet and keep them aside, then reheat the pan with butter.

5. Add the asparagus to the pan and cover it with a lid.

6. Cook until tender-crisp, 4 to 6 minutes, and serve with the lamb.

Nutrition Information: 380 calories, 18.5g of fat, 48g of protein, 4.5g of

carbohydrates, 2.5g of fiber, 2g of net carbohydrates

2. Kebabs of Lemon Chicken with Vegetables

Servings: 4 Servings

Prep time: 10 minutes

Cook time: 15 minutes

Ingredients:

- 1 pound of boneless thighs of meat, sliced into cubes

- 1/4 cup of olive oil

- 2 teaspoons lemon juice

- 1 teaspoon of garlic minced

- Salt and pepper

- 1 big yellow onion, diced into 2-inch parts

- 1 big red pepper, sliced into 2-inch parts

- 1 big green pepper, sliced into 2-inch fragments

Instructions:

1. Mix the olive oil, lemon juice, garlic, salt, and pepper with the chicken.

2. With the onion and peppers, slide the chicken onto skewers.

3. Preheat a grill and grease the grates on medium-high flame.

4. Grill the skewers from both sides for 2 to 3 minutes until the chicken is cooked.

Nutrition information: 360 calories, 21g of fat, 34g of protein, 8g of carbohydrates,

2g of fiber, 6g of net carbohydrates.

3.   Spicy Chicken Enchilada Casserole
Servings: 6 Servings

Prep Time: Fifteen minutes

Cook time: 1 hour

Ingredients:

- 2 pounds of boneless thighs of meat, sliced

- Salt and pepper

- 3 cups of salsa tomatoes

- 1 1/2 cups cheddar cheese shredded

- 3/4 cup of whipped cream

- 1 cup of diced avocado

- **Instructions:**

1. Preheat the oven to 375 F and grease a tray with a casserole.

2. Season the chicken with pepper and salt and spread it over the plate.

3. Spread the tomato salsa on the chicken and sprinkle the cheeses.

4. Cover the tray tightly with foil, and bake until the chicken is cooked, for 60 minutes.

5. Enjoy sour cream and sliced avocado.

Nutrition Information: 550 calories, 31.5g of fat, 54g of protein, 12g of carbohydrates, 4g of fiber, 8g of net carbohydrates

4. White Cheddar Broccoli Chicken Casserole
Servings: 6 Servings:

Prep Time: 15 minutes

Cook time: 30 minutes

Ingredients:

- 2 teaspoons of olive oil

- 1 pound boneless thighs of meat, chopped

- 1 yellow medium onion, chopped

- 1 garlic clove, minced

- 1 1⁄2 cups Chicken broth

- Cream cheese 8 ounces, melted

- 1/4 cup of sour cream

- 2 and a half cups of broccoli florets

- 3⁄4 cup of white cheddar cheese sliced

Instructions:

1. Preheat the oven to 350 F and grease a tray with a casserole.

2. Heat oil over medium-high flame in a large skillet.

3. Add the chicken and cook till golden brown for 2 to 3 minutes.

4. Stir in the garlic and onion, then season with salt and pepper.

5. Sauté for 4 to 5 minutes before the chicken is thoroughly cooked.

6. Mix the chicken broth into the mixture, then add the cream cheese and sour cream.

7. Simmer until it is melted with the cream cheese, then stir in the broccoli.

8. In the casserole bowl, pour the mixture and sprinkle it with cheese.

9. Bake until hot and bubbly, for 25 to 30 minutes.

Nutrition Information: 435 calories, 32g of fat, 29.5g of protein, 6g of

carbohydrates, 1.5g of fiber, 4.5g of net carbohydrates

5.   Stuffed Bell Peppers Bacon
Servings: 4 Servings

Prep Time: Fifteen minutes

Cook time: 45 minutes

Ingredients:

- 1 cauliflower, medium head, chopped

- 1 tablespoon of olive oil

- 12 ounces' Italian ground sausage

- 1 tiny yellow, chopped onion

- 1 dried oregano teaspoon

- Salt and pepper

- 4 medium peppers of the bell

Instructions:

1. Preheat the oven to 350°F.

2. Finely chop the cauliflower into rice-like grains in a food processor.

3. Heat the oil over medium heat in a pan, then Cook the cauliflower until tender.

4. Keep the cauliflower rice aside, then reheat the skillet.

5. Add the sausage and fry, also drain the fats once it's done.

6. Stir in the cauliflower with the bacon, mix the cabbage, oregano, salt, and pepper.

7. Slice off the pepper's tops, remove the seeds and pith and pour a little amount of mixture in it.

8. In a baking dish, put the peppers upright, then cover the platter with foil.

9. Bake for 30 minutes, then uncover it and bake for another 15 minutes. Serve it

hot.

Nutrition Information: 355 calories, 23.5g of fat, 19g of protein, 16.5g of carbohydrates, 6g of fiber, 10.5g total carbohydrates

5.4. Keto dessert recipes

1.   Cashew Macadamia Fat Bomb Bars
Servings: 16

Prep Time: 10 minutes

Cook Time: None

Ingredients:

- 1/2 cup of almond butter

- 1/4 cup of unsweetened cocoa powder

- 1/4 cup of erythritol powder

- 2 cups of sliced macadamia nuts

- 1/2 cup of heavy cream

Instructions:

1. In a shallow saucepan over a low fire, melt the almond butter.

2. Whisk in the cocoa powder and sweeten it with erythritol.

3. Stir in the heavy cream and sliced macadamia nuts until well mixed.

4. Pour the mixture into silicone molds and let them cool.

5. Place the molds into the fridge and refrigerate until they harden.

6. Pop out the fat bombs from molds and store them in an airtight jar.

Nutrition Info: 185 calories, 19.5g of fat, 2.5g of protein, 4.5g of carbohydrates, 2.5g

of fiber, 2g of net carbohydrates.

2. Coconut Truffles from Cocoa
Servings: 12 Servings:

Prep Time: Fifteen minutes

Time for Cook: Zero

Ingredients:

- 1 bottle of coconut butter
- 6 teaspoons of unsweetened ground cocoa
- 2 teaspoons of shredded coconut unsweetened
- 2 teaspoons Instant coffee powder
- Liquid extract of stevia, to taste
- 2 teaspoons of molten coconut oil

Instructions:

1. In the microwave, warm the coconut butter and stir until smooth.

2. Stir in the chocolate, coconut, stevia, and coffee powder.

3. Grease the ice cube tray with molten coconut oil.

4. Spoon the mixture of coconut chocolate into the ice cube tray and pat it flat.

5. Freeze for 4 hours or until firm, then defrost 15 minutes before serving.

Nutrition information: 290 calories, 28g of fat, 3.5g of protein, 11g of

 carbohydrates, 8g of fiber, 3g of net carbohydrates.

3.   Chocolate Sun butter
Servings: 16 Servings:

Time to prep: 5 minutes

Time for Cook: Zero

Ingredients:

- 1 cup of coconut oil

- 1 cup of butter of sunflower seed

- 1/2 cup of unsweetened cocoa powder

- 1/4 cup of coconut flour

- Liquid extract of stevia, to taste

Instructions:

1. In a small pan, melt the coconut oil and sunflower seed butter together.

2. Whisk together the coconut flour, ¼ cocoa powder, and Stevia liquid to taste.

3. Remove from the heat and allow to cool until slightly hardened.

4. Divide it into 16 pieces and roll it into balls and put it in a dish.

5. Coat the fat bombs with remaining cocoa powder and chill.

Nutrition information: 230 calories, 22g of fat, 4g of protein, 8g of carbohydrates,

2g of fiber, 6g of net carbohydrates.

4.   Coco-Almond Bomb Bars of Fat
Servings: 12 Servings:

Prep time: 10 minutes

Time for Cook: Zero

Ingredients:

- 1/2 cup of peanut butter

- 1/4 cup of unsweetened cocoa powder

- 1/4 cup of erythritol powder

- 2 cups of toasted almonds, sliced

- 1/2 cup of heavy cream

Instructions:

1. Melt the cocoa butter in a small saucepan over low heat.

2. Whisk in the cocoa powder and sweeten with erythritol.

3. Stir in the chopped almonds and heavy cream until well combined.

4. Pour the mixture into molds of silicone and let them cool.

5. Keep the molds in the fridge and refrigerate until they are hard.

6. Pop out the fat bombs from molds and store them in an airtight jar.

Nutrition Info: 205 calories, 20.5g fat, 4.5g protein, 5g carbs, 3g fiber, 2g

net carbohydrates

5.   Chocolate-Dipped Pecan Fat Bombs
Servings: 16 Servings:

Period for Prep: 10 minutes

Time for Cook: Zero

Ingredients:

- 1 bottle of coconut butter

- 1 cup canned coconut milk

- 1 cup finely chopped pecans

- 1 teaspoon vanilla extract

- Liquid extract of stevia, to taste

- ¼ cup chopped dark chocolate

- ½ teaspoon palm shortening

Instructions:

1. Mix the coconut butter and coconut milk in a small saucepan over low

   heat.

2. When the mixture melted, Stir in the pecans and vanilla, then add sweetener.

3. Remove from flame and chill for 1 to 2 hours until firm.

4. Divide the mixture into 16 pieces and make small balls.

5. Melt the dark chocolate in the microwave with the palm shortening.

6. Dip the balls in the chocolate and place them on a plate

7. Chill until the chocolate is hardened, then serve.

Nutrition Info: 245 calories, 24.5g fat, 3g protein, 9.5g carbs, 5.5g fiber, 4g net carbs

Conclusion

We have reached this juncture and I am so happy that you have selected to take the steps required on this ketogenic voyage. I hope, this book and its contents, will be able to give you step by step actionable value, for your efforts toward nutritional ketosis. More significantly, I hope that the book has also given you the self-confidence booster and has built up your promise to stay on the diet.

One of the main keys to any successful diet or lifestyle change has always been the choice of correct nutrients that fit in with the doctrines of the diet. Overall, eating moderate protein, rich fat, and low carbs might have an enormous influence on your health – dropping your body weight, cholesterol, blood sugar, and raising your mood levels and energy.

A ketogenic diet can be tough to fathom at the start but isn't as inflexible as it's made out to be. The alteration can be a little bit tough, but the increasing popularity of the clean eating program makes it easier and easier to find accessible low-carb foods. In the end, I would claim that this book is devoted to anyone who still unnecessarily trusts in traditional dietary advice, particularly if it has never helped them lose weight or get healthier and most definitely made things drastically worse.

Thanks a million, stay healthy and happy!

CPSIA information can be obtained
at www.ICGtesting.com
Printed in the USA
BVHW040802040321
R11947400001B/R119474PG601388BVX00006B/6